FOOD ADDITIVES
A Shopper's Guide To What's Safe
& What's Not

Christine Hoza Farlow, D.C.

2004 Revised Edition

KISS For Health Publishing, Escondido, California
"Keep It Simple Secrets For Health"

ISBN 0-9635635-5-6

This book is dedicated to all my patients, whose desire to improve their health through good nutrition inspired me to write this book, and to all people who are committed to better health without chemicals in their food.

Contents

HOW TO USE THIS BOOK

The codes below are to the left of each additive and indicate the safety of the additive.

*   GRAS - <u>G</u>enerally <u>R</u>ecognized <u>A</u>s <u>S</u>afe by the FDA.

φ   FDA approved colorant

S   There is no known toxicity. The additive appears to be safe.

A   The additive may cause allergic reactions.

C   Caution is advised. The additive may be unsafe, poorly tested, or used in foods we eat too much of.

C1   Caution is advised for certain groups in the population, such as pregnant women, infants, persons with high blood pressure, kidney problems, etc.

X   The additive is unsafe or very poorly tested.

The numbers below appear after some of the additives and indicate the purpose for which the additive is used, and the kinds of products in which you might find that additive.

1. <u>acidifier</u> - used in baked goods, candy, cheese, desserts, jelly, soft drinks.
2. <u>alkali</u> - used in baked goods, canned vegetables, chocolate, dairy products, frozen desserts, olives, tomato products.
3. <u>antibrowning agent</u> - used on fruits and vegetables.
4. <u>anticaking agent</u> - used in baking powder, nondairy creamer, salt, soft drink powders.
5. <u>antifoaming agent</u> - used in baked goods, beer, coffee creamer, fruit juices, jelly, dairy products, wine.
6. <u>antimycotic agent</u> - used in baked goods, cheese, dried fruit, jelly, processed meats, syrup.
7. <u>antioxidant</u> - used in bacon, baked goods, breakfast bars, butter, candy, canned fruits and vegetables, cream, fried foods, gelatin desserts, margarine, nuts, peanut butter, powdered soups, oil, salad dressing, shortening, spices, whipped toppings, foods containing artificial color or flavor.
8. <u>antistaling agent</u> - used in baked goods.
9. <u>artificial flavoring</u> - used in processed foods.
10. <u>artificial color</u> - used in baked goods, butter, cereal, candy, cheese, gelatin desserts, icing, maraschino

cherries, margarine, meat, oranges, pasta, pudding, soft drinks.

11. <u>artificial sweetener</u> - used in processed foods.
12. <u>binder</u> - used in processed foods, snack foods.
13. <u>bleaching agent</u> - used in baked goods, cheese, fats, flour, oils.
14. <u>buffer</u> - used in baked goods, canned vegetables, cereals, cheese, chocolate, dessert mixes, jelly, ham, ice cream, pasta, soft drinks, syrups.
15. <u>clarifying agent</u> - used in beer, soft drinks, vinegar, wine.
16. <u>color preservative</u> - used in processed foods.
17. <u>crystallization inhibitor</u> - used in oil and sugar products.
18. <u>dough conditioner</u> - used in baked goods.
19. <u>emulsifier</u> - used in baked goods, cake mixes, candy, chocolate, dairy products, ice cream, margarine, nondairy creamer, peanut butter, pickles, processed meats, shortening, toppings.
20. <u>enzymes</u> - used in cheese, fats, hydrolyzed protein.
21. <u>fat substitute</u> - used in dairy-type products, fried foods, frozen desserts, low fat products, margarine, mayonnaise.
22. <u>filler</u> - used in processed foods.
23. <u>firming agent</u> - used on fruits and vegetables.
24. <u>flavor carrier</u> - used in candy, soft drinks, syrups.
25. <u>flavor & color solvent</u> - used in coffee decaffeination, herbs, spices.

26. <u>flavor enhancer</u> - used in canned vegetables, fruit drinks, gelatin desserts, gravy, ice cream, jelly, meat products, nondairy creamer, sauces, soft drinks, soups, soup mixes.
27. <u>flavoring agent</u> - used in processed foods.
28. <u>foaming agent</u> - used in frozen desserts.
29. <u>food coating/glaze</u> - used in candy, on fruits and vegetables.
30. <u>food grade shellac</u> - used on candy.
31. <u>fungus source of enzymes</u> - used in baked goods, beef.
32. <u>humectant</u> - used in baked goods, candy, diet food, ice cream, jelly, shredded coconut, soft drinks.
33. <u>leavening</u> - used in baked goods, brewed drinks, cake mixes, flour.
34. <u>maturing agent</u> - used in baked goods.
35. <u>meat tenderizer</u>
36. <u>milk protein</u>
37. <u>milk sugar</u>
38. <u>natural food color</u> - see artificial color.
39. <u>neutralizer</u> - used in dairy products, processed foods.
40. <u>preservative</u> - used in processed foods.
41. <u>propellant gas</u> - used in whipping cream, vegetable sprays.
42. <u>protein extender</u> - used in processed foods.
43. <u>salt substitute</u>
44. <u>sequestrant</u> - used in beverages, fats, oils.
45. <u>softener</u> - used in processed foods.

46. <u>stabilizer</u> - used in baked goods, cocoa, fruit drinks, ice cream, pudding.
47. <u>stimulant</u> - in chocolate, cocoa, coffee, soft drinks.
48. <u>suspending agent</u> - used in processed foods.
49. <u>sweetener</u> - used in processed foods.
50. <u>texturizer</u> - used in canned goods, frozen desserts, ice cream, other processed foods.
51. <u>thickener</u> - used in baby food and formula, ice cream, jelly, pudding, salad dressing, soft drinks, soup, yogurt.
52. <u>yeast food</u> - used in baked goods, beer, wine; may contain free glutamates.

WHY YOU SHOULD USE THIS BOOK

This book will guide you when you're shopping to help you make informed choices about the foods you buy. It's purposely small so you can carry it in your pocket or purse.

There are more than 3000 different chemicals that are purposefully added to our food supply. The testing for the safety of these chemical additives is generally done by the company that wants to produce the chemicals or to use the chemical additives in the foods they produce. The Delaney Clause of the 1958 Food Additives Amendment states that any additives shown to cause cancer in humans or animals are not permitted to be added to our food. However, political pressure has caused the FDA to relax these standards and allow small amounts of cancer causing substances to be used in foods.

Even if all of the food additives used in our foods were safe individually, rarely does any food have only one additive in it. Testing for additive safety has been done for individual additives, not for combinations of additives. Additives that are safe individually may be harmful in certain combinations. **Nobody knows the effects of the many different additives used in the thousands of different combinations.**

This book lists 800 of the most common food additives. Each additive is preceded by a code representing its safety and the advisability of its use. The code indicates if the additive is generally recognized as safe (GRAS) by the FDA, and an evaluation of its safety and advisability of its use, *independent of the FDA evaluation.* The codes are listed on page 7 under **HOW TO USE THIS BOOK**.

The GRAS classification of safety by the FDA does not guarantee that the additive is safe. The FDA evaluates additives based upon their ability to cause cancer and harmful reproductive effects, generally ignoring other harmful outcomes. In addition, a number of formerly GRAS additives have been removed from the GRAS list *after they were found to be harmful.* It is virtually certain that some additives in common use now, and considered to be safe, will one day be banned. For more information, see the bibliography at the end of the book.

Some of the additives are followed by a number or series of numbers. These numbers represent a code for the uses of the additives. These codes are listed on pages 8 - 11.

The additive listing may also include some of the adverse effects that may be associated with consumption of the additive, and if the additive has not been adequately tested.

HOW TO READ LABELS

Finding the ingredients on the label and being able to read them can be a challenge. They are often hidden under a flap of packaging material in very tiny print, barely readable without a magnifying glass.

Often the package has statements like "NATURAL FRUIT FLAVORS, with Real Fruit Juice," or ALL NATURAL INGREDIENTS and NO PRESERVATIVES ADDED. This **DOES NOT** mean there are no harmful additives in the product. The manufacturer hopes you'll think these are healthy, natural products, but if you read the list of ingredients and compare each additive with the additives listed in this book, you'll see it's not true.

Ingredients are listed on the label in order of predominance by weight...the ingredient that weighs the most is listed first, the ingredient that weighs the least is listed last.

Here's a general rule of thumb: if the list of ingredients is long, there's probably a lot of chemical additives in the product, and you're risking your health by eating it. If the list of ingredients is short, it may or may not have harmful additives in it, so read the ingredients carefully before you decide to purchase the product.

Nutrition Facts gives you information on calories, and grams of fat, cholesterol, sodium, carbohydrates, dietary fiber, sugars, and protein in each serving. Here's some useful conversions to help you use and understand this information better.

1 gram of fat = approximately 9 calories.
1 gram of protein = approximately 4 calories.
1 gram of carbohydrate = approximately 4 calories.
4 grams of sugar = 1 teaspoon of sugar.

Let's take an example of a 123 calorie snack with 7 grams of fat, 2 grams of protein and 13 grams of carbohydrate of which 12 grams of the carbohydrate is sugar.

To get fat calories, multiply 9x7=63 calories from fat.
To get percentage of fat, divide 63 fat calories by 123 snack calories to get 51% fat.

Use the same procedure for protein and carbohydrate, using 4 calories per gram instead of 9.

To get the number of teaspoons of sugar in the snack, divide 12 grams of sugar in the snack by 4, to get 3 teaspoons of sugar.

$$\frac{12 \text{ grams of sugar}}{4 \text{ grams per teaspoon}} = 3 \text{ teaspoons of sugar}$$

The example is summarized below.

	grams	calories	Percent
Fat	7	63	51%
Protein	2	8	7%
carbohydrate (total)	13	52	42%
sugar	12	48	39%
other	1	4	3%

Buying a packaged product in a health food store does not guarantee that it will be free of harmful additives. The only way to be sure there are no harmful additives in the food you buy is to read every label of every package and buy fresh, whole organic foods whenever possible.

HOW TO IDENTIFY
GENETICALLY MODIFIED PRODUCE

If you're eating non-organically grown food, you're probably eating some genetically modified food without even knowing it. Genetically modified food has been on the marketplace for some time now. It's not labeled and it doesn't appear that labeling will be required anytime in the near future.

You can, however, tell if the fresh fruits and vegetables you buy have been genetically modified by those irritating little stickers that they put on the produce. If the item does not have a sticker on it, just look at the sign for a 4 or 5-digit number.

If the number is:

> 4 digits, it's conventionally grown.
> 5 digits starting with 9, it's organically grown.
> 5 digits starting with 8, it's genetically modified

At this time, there is no way of knowing if the ingredients in packaged or canned foods have been genetically modified, unless they're organic. Organically grown foods are not genetically modified.

FOOD ADDITIVES

* C A   <u>Acacia gum</u> - 17, 19, 46; may cause skin rashes; not adequately tested.

  X   <u>Acesulfame-K</u> - 11, "Sunette"; may cause low blood sugar attacks; causes cancer, elevated cholesterol in lab animals; not adequately tested.

  X   <u>Acesulfame-potassium</u> - same as acesulfame-K.

  C A <u>Acetal</u> - may cause breathing difficulty, heart problems, high blood pressure; central nervous system depressant.

* C   <u>Acetaldehyde</u> - 9; irritant to mucous membranes, central nervous system depressant, large doses may cause death.

  C   <u>Acetate</u> - 27; may cause stomach irritation in large amounts.

* C   <u>Acetic acid</u> - 1, 27; may cause gastrointestinal distress, skin rashes, eye irritation.

* S   <u>Acetoin</u> - 27.

  C   <u>Acetone peroxide</u> - 13, 34, not adequately tested.

* S   <u>Acetyl methylcarbinol</u> - 27.

  C A <u>Acetylated mono- and diglycerides</u> - 19, see mono- & diglycerides.

* S   <u>Aconitic acid</u> - 27.

* S   <u>Adiptic acid</u> - 1, 27, 40.

* C A <u>Agar-agar</u> - 17, 32, 46, 51; may cause flatulence, bloating; may have laxative effect.

  C   <u>Aguamiel</u> - 49; derived from cactus; use

sparingly.

S A Albumins - 46, 50, 51; may be egg, milk based.
* S Alfalfa - 27.
* Cl Alginates - 17, 28, 46, 50; possible pregnancy complications.
* Cl Alginic acid - 5, 46; may cause birth defects.
C Alitame – 11; related to aspartame; not adequately tested; awaiting approval.
X A Alkyl gallate - may cause liver problems.
C Alkyl sulfates - may cause skin rashes.
* S Allspice - 27.
* C Allyl isothiocyanate - 27; toxic; may cause skin problems.
C A Allyl sulfide - may cause breathing difficulty, kidney, liver problems.
* C Almond oil - 27; very toxic if not distilled to remove hydrocyanic acid; nontoxic if distilled.
C Aloe extract - may cause gastrointestinal distress, kidney problems.
* S A Alpha tocopherol - vitamin E; may be corn, peanut, soy based; see alpha tocopherol acetate.
S Alpha tocopherol acetate - vitamin E; large doses may be harmful if high blood pressure; see nutrient additives.
C Alum - see aluminum.
C Aluminum - may be associated with senility, memory problems, kidney problems, neurological problems, mouth ulcers, mineral

19

malabsorption; not adequately tested.

* C   <u>Aluminum ammonium sulfate</u> - 4; may cause vomiting; see aluminum, ammonium.
* C   <u>Aluminum calcium silicate</u> - 4; see aluminum.
  C   <u>Aluminum chloride</u> - see aluminum.
* C   <u>Aluminum hydroxide</u> - 33; may cause constipation; see aluminum.
  C   <u>Aluminum nicotinate</u> - may cause gastrointestinal distress; see aluminum, niacin.
* C   <u>Aluminum potassium sulfate</u> - may cause gastrointestinal distress; see aluminum.
* C   <u>Aluminum silicate</u> - 51; has caused death in lab animals; see aluminum.
* C   <u>Aluminum sodium sulfate</u> - see aluminum.
* C   <u>Aluminum sulfate</u> - see aluminum.
  C   <u>Amasake</u> - 49; may contain aspergillus oryzae, a suspected carcinogen.
 X A   <u>Ammonia</u> - corrosive; toxic if inhaled; eye and mucous membrane irritant; can burn eyes and skin; can cause permanent damage; may cause mouth ulcers, nausea, kidney, liver problems.
* C   <u>Ammonium alginate</u> - see ammonia, alginates.
* C   <u>Ammonium bicarbonate</u> - 33; may cause gastrointestinal distress; see ammonia.
* C   <u>Ammonium carbonate</u> - see ammonia.
  C   <u>Ammonium carrageenan</u> - see ammonia, carrageenan.
 C A   <u>Ammonium caseinate</u> - 50; see ammonia,

casein.

* X   <u>Ammonium chloride</u> - may cause gastrointestinal distress; toxic if ingested in large amounts; may cause irreversible damage; see ammonia.

* C   <u>Ammonium citrate</u> - 23, 26, 44; see ammonia.

* X A   <u>Ammonium glutamate</u> - 26; see ammonia, MSG.

   C   <u>Ammonium hydrogen carbonate</u> - ammonium bicarbonate; see ammonia.

* C   <u>Ammonium hydroxide</u> - see ammonia.

* C   <u>Ammonium isovalerate</u> - see ammonia.

* C   <u>Ammonium phosphate</u> - see ammonia phosphates.

* C   <u>Ammonium sulfate</u> - 18; see ammonia.

   X A   <u>Ammonium sulfite</u> - 7, 40; see sodium bisulfite.

   C   <u>Amyl acetate</u> - 27; may cause central nervous system depression, headaches, fatigue, mucous membrane irritation.

   X   <u>Amyl alcohol</u> - 27; highly toxic, has caused deaths.

   S A   <u>Amylases</u> – 18; may be soy based, genetically modified.

* C A   <u>Anethole</u> - 9; may cause mouth ulcers, burning sensation in mouth.

* C A   <u>Angelica</u> - may cause sensitivity to light.

   C   <u>Animal or vegetable shortening</u> - associated with heart disease, hardening of the arteries, elevated cholesterol levels.

φ S   <u>Annatto</u> - 27, 38.

C A   <u>Arabinogalactan</u> - 12, 19, 46, 51; not adequately tested.

S   <u>Arrowroot</u> – no known toxicity.

X   <u>Artemisia</u> - 27; may cause headaches, nervous system irritation, gastrointestinal distress, coma, death in large amounts.

X A   <u>Artificial color FD & C, U.S certified food color</u> contribute to hyperactivity in children; may contribute to learning and visual disorders, nerve damage; may be carcinogenic; see FD&C Colors.

C A   <u>Artificial flavoring</u> – may contain MSG or HVP; may cause reproductive disorders, developmental problems; not adequately tested.

C   <u>Artificial sweeteners</u> - associated with health problems; see specific sweetener.

S A   <u>Ascorbates</u> - 7; may be corn based; see ascorbic acid.

* S A   <u>Ascorbic acid</u> - 1, 7; synthetic vitamin C; see nutrient additives; can enhance mineral absorption, can inhibit nitrosamine formation; may be corn based.

* S   <u>Ascorbyl palmitate</u> - 7, see ascorbic acid.

X   <u>Aspartame</u> - 11; may cause brain damage in phenylketonurics; may cause central nervous system disturbances, menstrual difficulties; may affect brain development in unborn fetus.

C   <u>Aspergillus oryzae</u> - 29; may be carcinogenic.

X A   <u>Azo dyes</u> - 10; may cause gastrointestinal distress, nausea, hay fever, itching, high blood pressure; see artificial color....

C   <u>Azodicarbonamide</u> - 34; not adequately tested.

S   <u>Azulene</u> - naturally occuring plant compound found in chamomile tea.

S   <u>Bakers yeast glycan</u> - 19, 46, 51.

S   <u>Bakers yeast protein</u> - 33.

C A   <u>Baking powder</u> - 18, may contain corn; double acting may contain aluminum.

* C   <u>Baking soda</u> - see sodium bicarbonate.

C   <u>Banana oil</u> - see amyl acetate.

C   <u>Barbados molasses</u> - 49; see sucrose.

C   <u>Barley malt</u> - 49; 1 Tbsp. contains 6 grams of sugar; better tolerated by people with blood sugar disorders, all sweeteners best avoided, may contain free glutamates; see sucrose, MSG.

* S A   <u>Beeswax</u> - 19, 27, 29.

φ S   <u>Beet powder</u> – 38.

* C   <u>Bentonite</u> - 51; see aluminum silicate.

* C   <u>Benzaldehyde</u> - 9; may cause central nervous system depression, decreased sex drive, immune system stress.

* C A   <u>Benzoate of soda</u> - 40; can cause skin rashes, gastrointestinal upset, hyperactivity in children, neurological disorders; has caused birth defects in lab animals; moderately toxic if

swallowed; those with asthma or liver problems should avoid.

* C A   <u>Benzoic acid</u> - 6, 40, see benzoate of soda.

* C   <u>Benzoic aldehyde</u> - 9; see benzaldehyde.

* C   <u>Benzoyl peroxide</u> - 13, 18; destroys vitamin A, C, E, may cause skin rashes.

  C   <u>Benzyl acetate</u> - 27; may cause gastrointestinal upset.

  C   <u>Benzyl acetoacetate</u> - 27; see benzyl acetate.

  C   <u>Benzyl alcohol</u> - 9; may cause diarrhea, vomiting; see benzaldehyde.

  C   <u>Benzyl ethyl ether</u> - 27; narcotic in large amounts.

  C   <u>Benzyl formate</u> - 27; narcotic in large amounts.

  C   <u>Bergamot</u> - 27; may cause sensitivity to light.

* S   <u>Beta Carotene</u> - 38; precursor to vitamin A; see nutrient additives.

  S   <u>Beta glucans</u> – acomponent of cellulose.

* X A   <u>BHA</u> - 7, 40; can cause liver and kidney damage, behavioral problems, infertility, weakened immune system, birth defects, cancer; should be avoided by infants, young children, pregnant women and those sensitive to aspirin.

* X A   <u>BHT</u> - 7; see BHA; banned in England.

  C   <u>Blackstrap molasses</u> - 49; 1 Tbsp. contains 11-15 grams of sugars; contains small amounts of minerals, but is still 65% sucrose.

* S   <u>Biotin</u> - B vitamin; see nutrient additives.

C   Biphenyl - may cause nausea, vomiting, eye, nose irritation.

X A   Blue No. 1 - see FD&C Blue No. 1.

X A   Blue No. 2 - see FD&C Blue No. 2.

X   Boric acid - highly toxic; ingestion and topical application have caused poisoning.

C   Borneol - 27; may cause gastrointestinal disturbances, dizziness, convulsions.

X   Bromated flour – see potassium bromate.

X A   Brominated vegetable oil - 19, 24; has caused death in lab animals; stored in body fat; linked to major organ system damage, birth defects, growth problems; on FDA suspect list; banned in Belgium, Sweden and Great Britain.

C   Broth – see free glutamates.

* C   Brown algae - Possible mercury contamination; avoid during pregnancy; not adequately tested.

S   Brown rice syrup - 49; 1 Tbsp. contains 5 grams of sugars; better tolerated by people with blood sugar disorders, all sweeteners are best avoided, see sucrose.

C   Butane - 41; see isobutane.

* C   Butanoic acid - 27; has caused cancer in animals.

C   Butyl acetate - 9; may cause eye irritation; see benzaldehyde.

C   1,3 butylene glycol - 24, 32; may cause gastrointestinal upset, nervous system disorders.

* X A   Butylated hydroxyanisole - see BHA.

* X A   <u>Butylated hydroxytoluene</u> - see BHT.
    C   <u>Butylparaben</u> - 6, 40, aspirin sensitive should avoid, not adequately tested.
    C   <u>Butyraldehyde</u> - 9; ingredient in rubber cement.
    C   <u>Butyric acid</u> - 27; see butanoic acid.
   X A   <u>BVO</u> - see brominated vegetable oil.
* C   <u>Caffeine</u> - 47; psychoactive, addictive drug; may cause headaches, irritability, fertility problems, increases risk of miscarriage, birth defects, heart disease, depression, nervousness, behavioral changes, insomnia, etc., inhibits fetal growth.
* C   <u>Calcium acetate</u> - 44; low oral toxicity.
* C1   <u>Calcium alginate</u> - 50; see alginates.
* S A   <u>Calcium ascorbate</u> - 7; see ascorbic acid.
   C A   <u>Calcium benzoate</u> - see benzoate of soda.
    C   <u>Calcium bromate</u> - 34; see potassium bromate.
* S   <u>Calcium carbonate</u> - 2, 24, 39, 52; see nutrient additives; may constipate.
   C A   <u>Calcium caseinate</u> - 50; may contain free glutamates; see casein, MSG.
* C   <u>Calcium chloride</u> - 23; see nutrient additives; may cause heart problems, gastrointestinal upset.
* S A   <u>Calcium citrate</u> - 14, 18, 44; may interfere with results of medical lab tests, see nutrient additives; may be corn based.
* C   <u>Calcium diacetate</u> - 44; low oral toxicity.
   C A   <u>Calcium disodium EDTA</u> - 7, 44; see EDTA.
    C   <u>Calcium formate</u> - may cause urinary tract

problems.

S A   <u>Calcium fumarate</u> - 1; may contain corn.

* C A   <u>Calcium gluconate</u> - 14, 23, 26, 44; may cause gastrointestinal upset, heart problems; may be corn sugar based.

* S   <u>Calcium glycerophosphate</u> - see nutrient additives.

* C   <u>Calcium hexametaphosphate</u> - 19, 44, 50; see calcium phosphate.

* C   <u>Calcium hydroxide</u> - 23; lye, skin irritant.

* C1A   <u>Calcium iodate</u> - 17, 18; caution if thyroid problems.

* C A   <u>Calcium lactate</u> - 3, 14, 23, 52; may cause cardiac or gastrointestinal disturbances; may be corn or milk based; see nutrient additives.

* S   <u>Calcium oxide</u> - 1, 18, 52; skin, mucous membrane irritant; see nutrient additives.

* S   <u>Calcium pantothenate</u> - vitamin B5; see nutrient additives.

C   <u>Calcium peroxide</u> - 13, 18; not adequately tested.

* C   <u>Calcium phosphate</u> - 13, 18, 50; see nutrient additives; may reduce mineral absorption; may cause kidney damage.

* C A   <u>Calcium propionate</u> – 6, 40; can trigger behavioral changes.

* S   <u>Calcium pyrophosphate</u> - see nutrient additives.

* C   <u>Calcium silicate</u> - 4; may cause kidney problems, possibility of asbestos contamination.

C	<u>Calcium sodium EDTA</u> - 7, 44; see EDTA.
* C	<u>Calcium sorbate</u> - 6, 40; see sorbic acid.
* C A	<u>Calcium stearate</u> - 4; may be corn, peanut, soy based; may be derived from hydrogenated oils.
C A	<u>Calcium stearoyl lactylate</u> - 18, 19, 46; may be corn, milk, peanut, soy based; may be derived from hydrogenated oils.
* C	<u>Calcium sulfate</u> - 18, 34; may constipate; can kill rodents; see nutrient additives.
X A	<u>Camphor oil</u> - 27; has caused fetal death in pregnant women; toxic effects in adults.
* S	<u>Candelilla wax</u> - 29.
X	<u>Canola oil</u> – toxic; genetically engineered from rapeseed oil; processed at extremely high temperatures; depletes body stores of vitamin E; contains trans fats; caused kidney, heart, thyroid and adrenal problems in lab animals; depresses the immune system; blocks enzyme function; no studies done on humans for safety.
ɸ C	<u>Canthaxanthin</u> - 38; not adequately tested.
C	<u>Caprenin</u> - 21; not adequately tested.
* S	<u>Caprylic acid</u> - 9.
* C	<u>Capsicum</u> - may cause gastrointestinal upset.
* C	<u>Caramel</u> - 27, 38; may be processed with caustic chemicals, sulfites or ammonia; on FDA list to be tested for teratogenic, mutagenic and reproductive effects; suspected carcinogen; may cause inflammation of the tongue, scalp lesions,

dandruff, hair loss.

* C   <u>Caramel color</u> – see caramel.

C   <u>Caramel color III</u> – processed with ammonia; causes reduced white blood count in lab animals and decreased immune functon.

C A   <u>Carbohydrate gum</u> – resins derived from the bark of plants; see acacia gum, guar gum, gum ghatti, gum karaya, gum tragacanth.

* S   <u>Carbon dioxide</u> - 41.

* C A   <u>Carboxymethylcellulose</u> - 4, 17, 19, 32, 46, 50, 51; causes cancer in animals; mild irritant to eyes, skin and respiratory tract.

φ C A   <u>Carmine</u> - 38; may cause hives, life-threatening allergic reactions; not adequately tested.

* C   <u>Carnauba wax</u> - 29; not adequately tested.

* C A   <u>Carob bean gum</u> - 18, 51; not adequately tested.

* S   <u>Carotene</u> - 38; see beta carotene.

C   <u>Carrageenan</u> - 19, 46, 51; undegraded carrageenan has not caused cancer in test animals; degraded carrageenan has caused cancer in rats; inadequate information to determine carcinogenicity in humans; product labels do not distinguish between degraded and undegraded carrageenan; possible carcinogen; may contain free glutamates; should not be given to infants; see MSG; on FDA list for further study.

C   <u>Carvacrol</u> - 9; essential oil; oregano oil; antimicrobial; therapeutic in very small amounts;

large amounts are corrosive and harmful if swallowed or inhaled and destructive of skin and mucous membranes; can cause circulatory/respiratory depression, heart failure; do not use if pregnant or nursing.

* C   Carvol - 9, 47; see d-carvone.

* C   d-carvone - 9; may be toxic in large amounts.

* C   l-carvone - 9; see d-carvone.

* C A   Casein - 36, 50, 51; harmful to anyone with milk allergies; may contain traces of LAL, a chemical of questionable safety.

   C A   Caseinates - cause kidney damage in rats.

* C A   Cassia oil - 9; can cause upper respiratory irritation.

   C A   Castor oil - 9; large amounts may cause pelvic congestion and induce abortion.

   C   Cayenne pepper - see capsicum.

   X   Cedar - 27; see camphor oil.

   C   Cedar leaf oil - may cause reproductive failure, sensitivity to light.

   X   Cedar wood oil - 27; see camphor oil.

   S   Cellulose - plant fiber

* C A   Cellulose gum - see carboxymethylcellulose.

   C   Chlorine dioxide - 13, 34; suspected carcinogen.

   S   Cholecalciferol - vitamin D3; see nutrient additives.

* S   Choline bitartrate - a vitamin; see nutrient additives.

* S   <u>Choline chloride</u> - a vitamin; see nutrient additives.
* C   <u>Chondrus extract</u> - 46; see carrageenan.
   C A   <u>Cinnamal</u> - see cinnamaldehyde.
* C A   <u>Cinnamaldehyde</u> - 9; may cause gastrointestinal irritation; irritant to skin and mucous membranes.
* C A   <u>Cinnamic aldehyde</u> - 9; see cinnamaldehyde.
* C A   <u>Cinnamon</u> - see cinnamaldehyde.
* C A   <u>Cinnamon bark extract</u> - may cause skin rashes.
* C A   <u>Cinnamon bark oil</u> - may cause skin rashes.
* C   <u>Citral</u> - 9; interferes with wound healing.
* S A   <u>Citric acid</u> - 1, 7, 27, 44; may erode tooth enamel; may be corn based; may contain free glutamates.
   X A   <u>Citrus Red No. 2</u> - see FD&C Citrus Red No. 2.
* C A   <u>Cloves</u> - 9; see cassia oil.
   C   <u>Clove bud oil</u> - 27; has caused gastrointestinal irritation in lab animals.
   C   <u>Clove leaf oil</u> - 27; see clove bud oil.
   C   <u>Clove stem oil</u> - 27; see clove bud oil.
* C   <u>Clover</u> - may cause sensitivity to light.
* C   <u>CMC</u> - see carboxymethylcellulose.
   X A   <u>Coal tar dyes</u> - 10; may cause hay fever, skin rashes, nausea, itching, gastrointestinal distress, high blood pressure; see artificial color....
φ C A   <u>Cochineal</u> - 38; see carmine.
* C   <u>Cocoa</u> - contains caffeine-like chemical; Dutch process cocoa processed with alkali; see caffeine.

* S   Coconut oil – helps the body metabolize fatty acids; substitute for butter; use for frying and baking; use only non-hydrogenated.

C   Coffee – possible carcinogen.

* C   Confectioner's glaze - 30; no studies evaluating safety in food use.

C   Copper carbonate - see copper salts.

C   Copper chloride - see copper salts.

* C   Copper gluconate - see copper salts.

C   Copper hydroxide - see copper salts.

C   Copper orthophosphate - see copper salts.

C   Copper oxide - see copper salts.

C   Copper pyrophosphate - see copper salts.

C   Copper salts - see nutrient additives; skin and mucous membrane irritants; can cause vomiting.

* C   Copper sulfate - most highly irritating copper salt; see copper salts.

* S A   Corn gluten - 42, 50.

C   Corn protein – see free glutamates.

* C   Corn silk - 27; not adequately tested.

* C A   Corn starch - 51; may cause hay fever, eye, nose irritation.

* C A   Corn sugar - see corn syrup.

* C A   Corn syrup – 49, 51; associated with blood sugar problems, depression, fatigue, B-vitamin deficiency, hyperactivity, tooth decay, periodontal disease, indigestion.

* Cl   Cream of tartar - 1, 4, 33; caution if kidney or

heart problems.

C   <u>Croscarmellose sodium</u> – see sodium carboxymethylcellulose.

C   <u>Crospovidone</u> – ingredient found in drugs and nutritional supplements; low toxicity; not considered a health hazard by the Joint FAO/WHO Expert Committee for Food Additives; safety testing data not available.

* C1A   <u>Cuprous iodide</u> - 17, 18; caution if thyroid problems.

S   <u>Cyanocobalamin</u> - vitamin B12; see nutrient additives.

X   <u>Cyclamates</u> - 11; banned; no longer believed to be carcinogenic, but increases the effect of other carcinogens; manufacturers petitioning FDA to rescind ban.

* S   <u>D-Pantothenyl alcohol</u> - see nutrient additives.

S   <u>Date sugar</u> - 49; 1 Tbsp. contains equivalent of 3 grams of sugars; all sweeteners best avoided.

* C A   <u>Datem</u> – see diacetyl tartaric acid esters of mono- & diglycerides.

S   <u>7-Dehydrocholesterol</u> - vitamin D3; see nutrient additives.

* C   <u>Decanal</u> – 9; moderately toxic if swallowed; eye and skin irritant.

S   <u>Devan Sweet</u> - 49; see rice syrup powder.

C   <u>Dextrans</u> - may be carcinogenic.

* C A   <u>Dextrin</u> - 17, 51; may be from wheat or corn.

* C A   <u>Dextrose</u> - 49; see corn syrup.
* C   <u>Diacetyl</u> - 9; not adequately tested.
* C A   <u>Diacetyl tartaric acid esters of mono- &</u>
       <u>diglycerides</u> - 19; see mono- & diglycerides.
* C A   <u>Diacylglycerol</u> – see mono- & diglycerides.
* C   <u>Dibasic ammonium phosphate</u> - see ammonium,
       phosphates.
* C   <u>Dibasic calcium phosphate</u> - see calcium
       phosphate.
* C   <u>Dibasic potassium phosphate</u> - see potassium
       phosphate.
* C   <u>Dicalcium phosphate</u> - see calcium phosphate.
  X   <u>Dichlorvos</u> – pesticide used on produce, flea
       collars, food packaging; possible carcinogen,
       teratogen.
* C A   <u>Diglycerides</u> - see mono- & diglycerides.
* S   <u>Dilauryl thiodipropionate</u> – 7; antioxidant.
* S   <u>Dill</u> - 27; can cause sensitivity to light.
  C   <u>Dill oil</u> - 27; potentially toxic in large amounts;
       use cautiously if epileptic.
  S   <u>Dillseed</u> - 27.
  C   <u>Dimethylpolysiloxane</u> - 5; possibility of asbestos
       contamination; may cause kidney problems.
  C   <u>Dioctyl sodium sulfosuccinate (DSS)</u> - 19, 46;
       laxative effect; may cause gastrointestinal
       irritation, birth defects; not adequately tested.
  C   <u>Diphenyl</u> - may cause nausea, vomiting, eye,
       nose irritation.

* C   <u>Dipotassium phosphate</u> - 14, 44; may reduce mineral absorption; may cause kidney damage.

C A   <u>Disodium guanylate</u> - 26; can aggravate gout; may be soy or yeast based; used in products containing MSG; not adequately tested.

C A   <u>Disodium inosinate</u> - 26; can aggravate gout; may be soy or yeast based; used in products containing MSG; not thoroughly tested.

* C   <u>Disodium phosphate</u> - 12, 14, 19, 44; can contribute to kidney problems, high blood pressure, fluid retention.

* C   <u>Disodium pyrophosphate</u> - see disodium phosphate.

S   <u>Disodium riboflavin phosphate</u> - vitamin B2; see nutrient additives.

C   <u>Dough conditioners</u> - reduce mineral availability.

C   <u>DSS</u> - see dioctyl sodium sulfosuccinate.

C A   <u>Durkex oil</u> - 24, 29; refined, bleached, deodorized, partially hydrogenated oil. See hydrogenated vegetable oil.

C A   <u>EDTA</u> - 7, 44; may cause skin irritation, gastrointestinal upset, liver and kidney damage, mineral imbalances; may cause errors in results of medical lab tests; not adequately tested.

C   <u>Enzyme of aspergillus oryzae</u> - 31; may be carcinogenic.

* C   <u>Enzyme-modified fats</u> - 27; may contain free glutamates; see MSG.

C	<u>Epsom salts</u> - see magnesium sulfate.
X	<u>Equal</u> - 11; see aspartame.
S	<u>Ergocalciferol</u> - vitamin D2; see nutrient additives.
* S A	<u>Erythorbic acid</u> – 7, 16; may be corn based.
C	<u>Erythritol</u> – 26, 32, 44, 46, 49, 50, 51; better tolerated than other sugar alcohols; see sugar alcohols.
X A	<u>Erythrosine</u> - may cause overactive thyroid, sensitivity to light; see coal tar dyes.
C	<u>Ester gum</u> - 19, 27, 45; inadequate data on safety available.
* C	<u>Ethanal</u> - 9; see acetaldehyde.
C	<u>Ethoxylated mono- & diglycerides</u> - 18; not adequately tested.
* C	<u>Ethyl acetate</u> - 9; nervous system depressant; prolonged inhalation can cause kidney, liver damage; may contribute to secondary infection.
* C	<u>Ethyl alcohol</u> - fatal in large doses.
* S	<u>Ethyl butyrate</u> - 9.
* C	<u>Ethyl cellulose</u> - 12, 22; see carboxymethylcellulose.
* C	<u>Ethyl formate</u> - 6, 27; skin and mucous membrane irritant, narcotic in high concentrations.
S	<u>Ethyl heptanoate</u> - 9.
C A	<u>Ethyl maltol</u> - 26; may be corn or wheat based; may be carcinogenic.

C   <u>Ethyl methyl phenylglycidate</u> - 9; adversely affects nervous system in lab animals.

C A   <u>Ethyl propionate</u> - 9; see propionic acid.

* C   <u>Ethyl vanillin</u> - 9; skin irritant; may cause organ system   damage, cancer in lab animals; moderately toxic.

C A   <u>Ethylenediamine tetraacetic acid</u> - see EDTA.

φ X A   <u>FD&C Blue No. 1</u> - 10; may cause itching, low blood pressure; may be carcinogenic; not adequately tested; see artificial color....

φ X A   <u>FD&C Blue No. 1 Lake</u> - coal tar dye; carcinogen; may contain aluminum; see FD&C Colors, aluminum.

φ X A   <u>FD&C Blue No. 2</u> - 10; may cause itching, low blood pressure, brain tumors in lab animals; see artificial color....

φ X A   <u>FD&C Blue No. 2 Lake</u> - coal tar dye; potential carcinogen; may contain aluminum; see FD&C Colors, aluminum.

φ X   <u>FD&C Colors</u> – colors considered safe by the FDA for use in food, drugs and cosmetics; most of the colors are derived from coal tar and must be certified by the FDA not to contain more than 10ppm of lead and arsenic; certification does not address any harmful effects these colors may have on the body; most coal tar colors are potential carcinogens, may contain carcinogenic contaminants, and cause allergic reactions.

φ X A   <u>FD&C Citrus Red No. 2</u> - 10; carcinogenic; restricted to specific uses; see artificial color....

φ X A   <u>FD&C Green No. 3</u> - 10; may be carcinogenic; ee FD&C Colors.

φ X A   <u>FD&C Green No. 3 Lake</u> – may contain aluminum; see FD&C Green No. 3, aluminum.

φ X A   <u>FD&C Red No. 3</u> - 10; causes thyroid tumors in lab animals; FDA recommends banning use.

φ C A   <u>FD&C Red No. 40</u> - 10; see artificial color....

φ X A   <u>FD&C Red No. 40 Aluminum Lake</u> – may be contaminated with a carcinogen; see FD&C Colors, aluminum.

φ C A   <u>FD&C Yellow No. 5</u> - 10; may cause hay fever, gastrointestinal upset, skin rashes; avoid if aspirin sensitive; see artificial color....

φ X A   <u>FD&C Yellow No. 5 Lake</u> – may contain aluminum; see FD&C Yellow No. 5, aluminum.

φ X A   <u>FD&C Yellow No. 6</u> - 10; causes tumors in lab animals; contaminated with carcinogens; see artificial color....

φ X A   <u>FD&C Yellow No. 6 Lake</u> – may contain aluminum; see FD&C Yellow No. 6, aluminum.

* C   <u>Ferric ammonium citrate</u> - see nutrient additives, ammonium; not adequately tested.

* C   <u>Ferric chloride</u> - not adequately tested.

38

* C   <u>Ferric citrate</u> - see ferric chloride.

   C   <u>Ferric orthophosphate</u> - see nutrient additives; see ferric chloride.

* C   <u>Ferric phosphate</u> - see ferric chloride.

* C   <u>Ferric pyrophosphate</u> - see nutrient additives, ferric chloride.

* C   <u>Ferric sodium pyrophosphate</u> - see ferric chloride.

* C   <u>Ferric sulfate</u> - see ferric chloride.

* C   <u>Ferrous fumarate</u> - see nutrient additives, ferrous gluconate.

* C   <u>Ferrous gluconate</u> - 14, 23, 26, 44; see nutrient additives; may cause gastrointestinal disturbances; not adequately tested.

* C   <u>Ferrous lactate</u> - see nutrient additives, ferrous gluconate.

* C   <u>Ferrous sulfate</u> - see nutrient additives, ferrous gluconate.

   S   <u>Folacin</u> - folic acid; B vitamin; see nutrient additives.

   S   <u>Folic Acid</u> - B vitamin; see nutrient additives.

* C   <u>Food shellac</u> - see confectioner's glaze.

   C   <u>Food starch</u> - see starch.

  X A   <u>Formaldehyde</u> - 40; used in animal feed; carcinogen; causes DNA damage.

   C   <u>Formic acid</u> - 27; may cause urinary tract problems.

   S   <u>FOS</u> - 49; see fructooligosaccharides.

X A   <u>Free glutamates</u> - 26; may cause brain damage, especially in children; **always found in** autolyzed yeast, calcium caseinate, gelatin, glutamate, glutamic acid, hydrolyzed corn gluten, hydrolyzed protein, hydrolyzed soy protein, monopotassium glutamate, monosodium glutamate, pea protein, plant protein extract, sodium caseinate, textured protein, yeast extract, yeast food and yeast nutrient; **may be in** barley malt, boullion, broth, carrageenan, citric acid, enzymes, anything enzyme modified, anything fermented, flavors & flavorings, malt extract, malt flavoring, maltodextrin, natural flavors and flavorings, natural chicken flavoring, natural beef flavoring, natural pork flavoring, pectin, protease, protease enzymes, seasonings, soy protein, soy protein concentrate, soy protein isolate, soy sauce, soy sauce extract, stock, whey protein, whey protein concentrate, whey protein isolate, anything that is enzyme modified, fermented, protein fortified or ultrapasteurized and foods that advertise NO MSG, NO Added MSG or NO MSG Added; see MSG, processed free glutamates.

S   <u>Fructooligosaccharides</u> - 49; can be used by those with candida and blood sugar problems; may cause intestinal gas.

C A   <u>Fructose</u> - 49; 1 Tbsp. contains 12-15 grams of sugars; may be corn based; may cause gastrointestinal distress, elevated triglycerides; large amounts has caused tumors in mice.

C   <u>Fruit juice concentrate</u> - 49; 1 Tbsp. contains 5.5-8.5 grams of sugars; may contain fungicides and pesticides.

C   <u>Fruit pectin</u> - 19, 46, 51; may contain free glutamates.

* C A   <u>Fumaric acid</u> - 1, 27; may be corn based.

C   <u>Fungal protease from aspergillus oryzae</u> - see enzyme of aspergillus oryzae.

C A   <u>Furcelleran</u> - 19, 46; inadequately tested.

* S   <u>Garlic</u> - 27.

* C A   <u>Gelatin</u> - 17, 46, 51; may contain sulfur dioxide and/or free glutamates; cannot be determined if from BSE animals (i.e. animals with mad cow disease); see sulfur dioxide, MSG.

C A   <u>Gelatine</u> - see gelatin.

C   <u>Gellan gum</u> – 46, 51; eye, skin, mucus membrane and respiratory irritant; harmful if inhaled, swallowed or absorbed through skin; may cause diarrhea; not adequately tested.

C   <u>Genetically modified organisms</u> – genes are taken from one species of plant, animal or virus and inserted into another species in order to produce a desirable trait, such as disease resistant or hardier crops. No one knows the long-term effects of eating genetically modified foods.

Genetically modified foods are being sold now and they are not being labeled. Certified organic foods are the only foods guaranteed not to be genetically modified. Foods that may be genetically modified if they are not organic include: red and green bell peppers, canola oil, corn and corn products, hydrolyzed vegetable protein, lactose, lecithin, soybeans and soy products, flax, papayas, potatoes, tomatoes, squash, enzymes, dairy products, sunflower oil, pet food.

* C   <u>Geranial</u> - 9; see citral.

* S A   <u>Glucono delta-lactone</u> - 1, 33; may be corn based.

* S A   <u>Gluconolactone</u> - 1, 33; may be corn based.

C A   <u>Glucose</u> - 49, 51; may be corn based; associated with blood sugar problems, depression, fatigue, B-vitamin deficiency, hyperactivity, tooth decay, periodontal disease, indigestion.

C   <u>Glucuronolactone</u> – safe in small quantities; there is no research on the safety of the large quantities in energy drinks; should not be consumed with alcohol; not adequately tested.

X A   <u>Glutamates</u> - 26; see MSG.

* X A   <u>Glutamic acid</u> - 26, 43; see MSG.

* X A   <u>Glutamic acid hydrochloride</u> - 26; see MSG.

S A   <u>Gluten</u>

* C A   <u>Glycerin</u> - 8, 25, 32; may be corn, peanut or soy

based; may cause headaches, nausea, excess thirst, elevated blood sugar.

C   <u>Glycine</u> – mildly toxic.

* C A   <u>Glycerol</u> - see glycerin.

C   <u>Glycerol esters of wood resin</u> - see ester gum.

C   <u>Glyceryl abietate</u> - see ester gum.

* C   <u>Glyceryl monostearate</u> - 19, 45; may be lethal to lab animals in large doses.

* C   <u>Glyceryl triacetate</u> - 27, 45; may be lethal to lab animals in large doses.

C A   <u>GMP</u> - see disodium guanylate.

C   <u>Granular fruit source</u> - 49; 1 Tbsp contains 7.5 grams of sugars.

X A   <u>Green No. 3</u> - 10; see FD&C Green No. 3.

* S   <u>Ground limestone</u> - 27.

* C A   <u>Guar gum</u> - 46, 51; may cause nausea, gastrointestinal upset, bloating.

* C A   <u>Gum arabic</u> - see acacia gum.

S   <u>Gum benzoin</u> – 27; no known toxicity.

C   <u>Gum furcelleran</u> – 19, 46, 51; on FDA's list to be studied for mutagenic, teratogenic, subacute and reproductive effects; not adequately tested.

* C A   <u>Gum ghatti</u> - 19, 46; not adequately tested.

* C A   <u>Gum guaiac</u> – 7; not adequately tested.

* C A   <u>Gum karaya</u> - 19, 50; not adequately tested.

* C A   <u>Gum tragacanth</u> - 46, 51; can cause severe allergic reactions; not adequately tested.

* S   <u>Helium</u> - 41.

C   Heptanal - see acetaldehyde.

C A   Heptylparaben - 6, 40; pregnant women and those sensitive to aspirin should avoid; not adequately tested.

* C A High fructose corn syrup - see fructose, corn syrup.

C   Honey - 49; 1 Tbsp. contains 16-18 grams of sugars; may contain botulism spores; potentially harmful or fatal to children under 18 months.

C A   HPP - see hydrolyzed vegetable protein.

C A   HSH – see hydrogenated starch hydrolysate.

C A   HVP - see hydrolyzed vegetable protein.

* C   Hydrochloric acid - 14, 39; may cause irritation to mucus membranes, gastrointestinal distress.

* C   Hydrogen peroxide - 13, 40; suspected carcinogen.

C A   Hydrogenated starch hydrolysate - 11; may cause gastrointestinal distress.

C A   Hydrogenated vegetable oil - associated with heart disease, breast and colon cancer, atherosclerosis, elevated cholesterol.

C A   Hydrolyzed plant protein - see hydrolyzed vegetable protein.

C A   Hydrolyzed vegetable protein - 22, 26; may cause brain and nervous system damage in infants; high salt content; may be corn, soy, or wheat based. Contains free glutamates.

X A   <u>Hydroxyethyl cellulose</u> – 19, 48, 51; harmful if swallowed, inhaled and on skin contact, severe eye irritant, mutagenic.

C A   <u>Hydroxylated lecithin</u> - 7, 19; not adequately tested.

C   <u>Hydroxypropyl cellulose</u> - see carboxymethylcellulose.

C   <u>Hydroxypropyl methylcellulose</u> - see carboxymethylcellulose.

C A   <u>Imitation flavorings</u> - see artificial flavoring.

C A   <u>IMP</u> - see disodium inosinate.

X A   <u>Indigo carmine</u> - see coal tar dyes.

* S   <u>Inositol</u> - a vitamin; see nutrient additives.

* S   <u>Inulin</u> – a constituent of many herbs; dietary fiber; prebiotic; health promoting benefits for the intestinal tract; largte amounts may cause flatulence or gastrointestinal distress.

* C A   <u>Invert sugar</u> – 49; promotes dental caries; see glucose and fructose.

C A   <u>Ionone</u> – 9; caused swelling of liver cells in rats; eye, skin respiratory and digestive tract irritant; not adequately tested.

* C   <u>Iron, elemental</u> - see nutrient additives; least toxic form of iron used in foods.

C   <u>Iron, reduced</u> - see nutrient additives, elemental iron.

C A   <u>Irradiation</u> - destroys vitamins and minerals; may be carcinogenic.

C   Isoamyl acetate - 9; may cause headaches, fatigue, mucous membrane irritation.

* S A   Isoascorbic acid - 7; see erythorbic acid.

* C   Iso-butane - 41; animal carcinogen; may cause asphyxiation in large doses.

C A   Isolated soy protein - 22; highly processed; may contain free glutamates; may be contaminated with nitrites; see free glutamates.

C   Isomalt – 4, 32, 49;excessive consumption may cause gastrointestinal distress.

* S A   Isopropyl citrate - 1, 7, 44; may interfere with results of medical lab tests.

* C A   Karaya gum - may cause gastrointestinal distress, dermatitis, asthma.

C   Kola nut extract - 9; contains caffeine.

C   Lactitol – see sugar alcohols.

C   L-ascorbic acid - synthetic vitamin C; see nutrient additives; may cause diarrhea, kidney problems in large doses.

* S   L-cysteine - amino acid; see nutrient additives.

* S   L-cysteine monohydrochloride - amino acid; see nutrient additives.

S   L-lysine - amino acid; see nutrient additives.

S A   Lactalbumin - 46, 50, 51; derived from milk.

C A   Lactalbumin phosphate - 46, 50, 51; see phosphates.

* C   Lactase enzyme preparation from Kluyveromyces lactis – see free glutamates.

* S A   <u>Lactic acid</u> - 1, 6, 7, 14, 27; may be corn or milk based.

   S   <u>Lactoflavin</u> - vitamin B2; see nutrient additives.

   C   <u>Lactose</u> - 37; may cause gastrointestinal distress.

   C A   <u>Lactylic stearate</u> - see calcium stearoyl lactylate.

   C A   <u>Larch gum</u> - see arabinogalactan.

   C   <u>Leavening</u> - may contain aluminum, BHA/BHT or chemical preservatives.

* S A   <u>Lecithin</u> - 7, 17, 19, 46, 51; soy, corn, egg, or peanut based; may lower cholesterol.

   C A   <u>Levulose</u> - see fructose.

* C   <u>Licorice</u> - 27; may cause high blood pressure, muscle and nervous system disorders in large amounts; may have medicinal benefits for gastric ulcers.

* S A   <u>Linoleic acid</u> - may be corn, peanut, soy based.

   C   <u>Lipase</u> – may be genetically modified.

   C   <u>Liquid fruit source</u> - 49; 1 Tbsp. contains 11 grams of sugars.

* C A   <u>Locust bean gum</u> - see carob bean gum.

   C   <u>Lycasin</u> – see hydrogenated starch hydrosylate.

* C   <u>Mace/nutmeg</u> - toxic to nervous system in large doses, can cause hallucinations; East Indian nutmeg may cause liver cancer.

   C1   <u>Magnesium acetate</u> - 2, 4, 14, 39; magnesium is essential nutrient; potentially harmful if kidney problems.

* C1   <u>Magnesium carbonate</u> - 2, 4, 13, 34; see nutrient

additives; magnesium is essential nutrient; potentially harmful if kidney problems.

* C1   <u>Magnesium chloride</u> - 16, 23; see nutrient additives, magnesium carbonate.

  C1A <u>Magnesium fumarate</u> - 1; may be corn based; see magnesium acetate.

  C1   <u>Magnesium gluconate</u> - see nutrient additives, magnesium carbonate.

* C1   <u>Magnesium hydroxide</u> - 2; see nutrient additives, magnesium carbonate.

* C1   <u>Magnesium oxide</u> - 39; see nutrient additives, magnesium carbonate.

* C1   <u>Magnesium phosphate</u> - see nutrient additives, magnesium carbonate.

* C1   <u>Magnesium silicate</u> - 4; see magnesium acetate.

* C1   <u>Magnesium stearate</u> - see nutrient additives, magnesium carbonate.

* C1   <u>Magnesium sulfate</u> - see nutrient additives, magnesium carbonate.

* S A   <u>Malic acid</u> - 1, 27; may be corn based.

  S A   <u>Malt</u> - 27, 49; may contain corn, wheat, or vinegar.

* C   <u>Malt extract</u> - 27, 49; see barley malt.

* C   <u>Malt syrup</u> - 27, 49; see barley malt.

  C   <u>Malted barley</u> - see barley malt.

* C   <u>Maltitol</u> – 27, 32, 46, 49, 51; may cause gastrointestinal distress when consumed in large amounts.

* C A   Maltodextrin - 26, 50; a sugar, may be corn based; may contain free glutamates; see sucrose, MSG.
* C A   Maltol - 26; may be corn or wheat based; may be carcinogenic.
  C A   Maltose - 49; may be corn, soy, wheat based.
* S   Manganese chloride - see nutrient additives; manganese is essential mineral; harmful in large amounts.
* S   Manganese citrate - see nutrient additives, manganese chloride.
* S   Manganese gluconate - see manganese chloride.
* S   Manganese glycerophosphate - see manganese chloride.
* S   Manganese hypophosphite - see nutrient additives, manganese chloride.
  C   Manganese oxide - not adequately tested.
* S   Manganese sulfate - see manganese chloride.
* S   Manganous oxide - see nutrient additives.
  C A   Mannitol – 32, 49, 50; small amounts may cause gastrointestinal distress; may cause nausea, kidney problems; sugar, seaweed or corn based; not thoroughly tested.
  C   Maple syrup - 49; 1 Tbsp. contains 13 grams of sugars; contains healthful minerals; use sparingly.
  C A   Margarine – see hydrogenated vegetable oil.
  S   Menadione - vitamin K3; skin and mucous

	membrane irritant; see nutrient additives.
S	<u>Menaquinone</u> - vitamin K2; see nutrient additives.
C	<u>Methionine</u> - amino acid; use as additive requires additional study; see nutrient additives.
C	<u>Menthol</u> – nontoxic in concentrations less than 3%; irritant in concentrations above 3%; may cause nausea, vomiting, abdominal pain, coma in high concentrations.
* C	<u>Methylcellulose</u> - 46, 51; see carboxymethylcellulose.
* C	<u>Methyl ethyl cellulose</u> - see carboxymethylcellulose.
* C	<u>Methylparaben</u> - 6, 40; avoid if aspirin sensitive; not adequately tested.
C	<u>Methyl polysilicone</u> - see dimethylpolysiloxane.
C	<u>Methyl silicone</u> - 5; see dimethylpolysiloxane.
C1	<u>Microcrystalline cellulose</u> - 4, 21, 24, 50; derived from vegetable, cereal or wood; no tests done regrding safety for infants and young children. Infants and young children should avoid.
* C	<u>Mixed carbohydrase and protease enzyme product</u> – may contain free glutamates.
* C	<u>Modified cellulose gum</u> – see sodium carboxymethylcellulose.
* C A	<u>Modified food starch</u> - 4, 32, 51; processed with chemicals of questionable safety; not adequately tested.

C A   <u>Modified maltodextrin</u> - see modified food starch, maltodextrin.

C   <u>Molasses</u> - 49; see sucrose.

* C A   <u>Mono- & diglycerides</u> - 5, 8, 17, 18, 19, 46; may be soy, corn, peanut or fat based; hydrogenated oils; not adequately tested.

* C A   <u>Monoammonium glutamate</u> - 26; see MSG.

* C   <u>Monobasic ammonium phosphate</u> - see ammonium, phosphates.

* C   <u>Monobasic calcium phosphate</u> - 44; see calcium phosphate.

* C   <u>Monobasic potassium phosphate</u> - see potassium phosphate.

* C   <u>Monocalcium phosphate</u> - see calcium phosphate.

* S A   <u>Monoisopropyl citrate</u> - 44; may interfere with results of medical lab tests.

* C A   <u>Monopotassium glutamate</u> - 26; may cause nausea, gastrointestinal upset; see MSG.

* C A   <u>Monosodium glutamate</u> - 26; see MSG.

* C   <u>Monosodium phosphate</u> - 14, 19, 32; see phosphates.

* C   <u>Monosodium phosphate derivatives of mono- and diglycerides</u> - 19; see mono- and diglycerides.

* X A   <u>MSG</u> - 26; mutagen; may cause headaches, itching, nausea, brain, nervous system, reproductive disorders, high blood pressure;

pregnant, lactating mothers, infants, small children should avoid; allergic reactions common; **may be hidden in** infant formula, baby food, low fat and no-fat milk, candy, chewing gum, drinks, kosher food, protein bars, protein powder, protein drinks recommended for seniors, most processed foods, wine, waxes applied to fresh fruits and vegetables, over-the-counter medications, especially children's, binders and fillers for nutritional supplements, prescription and non-prescription drugs, IV fluids given in hospitals, chicken pox vaccine, live virus vacines, nasal spray flu vaccine; used in pesticides, fungicides and fertilizers; being sprayed on growing fruits and vegetables as a growth enhancer (AuxiGro); proposed for use on organic crops. See free glutamates, processed free glutamates.

* C   <u>Mustard oil</u> - 27; see allyl isothiocyanate.

* C A   <u>Mycoprotein</u> - meat substitute made from a mold-like fungus; may cause nausea, vomiting, diarrhea and cramps, hives, difficulty breathing and anaphylactic reactions; not adequately tested.

* C   <u>N-butane</u> - see isobutane.

* C   <u>N-Butyric acid</u> - 9; see butanoic acid.

   C   <u>Natamycin</u> - 6; antibiotic used in cheese.

   C A   <u>Natural flavors</u> - may be chemically extracted and processed and in combination with other food additives not required to be listed on the label; may contain free glutamates; see MSG.

X   Neotame – similar to aspartame; approved 2002; industry sources cite at least 100 studies on the safety of neotame, however a search of PubMed and the National Library of Medicine could not find any published studies related to the safety of neotame; not adequately tested.

* C   Neral - 9; see citral.

* S   Niacin - vitamin B3; see nutrient additives; may cause flushing.

* S   Niacinamide - vitamin B3; see nutrient additives.

* X   Nickel - may cause dermatitis; ingestion of large amounts of nickel salts may cause kidney damage, gastrointestinal upset, nervous depression; carcinogen.

X   Nickel sulfate - nickel salt; see nickel.

S   Nicotinamide - see niacin; nutrient additives.

S   Nicotinic acid - see niacin; nutrient additives.

* C   Nisin - 40; bacteriocin, a gene encoded antimicrobial peptide or GMO, derived from lactic acid in pasteurized cheese; not required to be listed on the label.

X   Nitrates - 6, 16; form powerful cancer-causing agents in stomach; can cause death; considered dangerous by FDA but not banned because they prevent botulism.

X   <u>Nitrites</u> - may cause headaches, nausea, vomiting, dizziness; known to cause cancer; see nitrates.

* S   <u>Nitrogen</u> - 41.

C   <u>Nitrosyl chloride</u> - 13, 34; irritant to skin, eyes, mucous membranes; inhalation may cause ulmonary edema and hemorrhage.

* Cl   <u>Nitrous oxide</u> - 41; has caused damage to fetus in pregnant lab animals.

* C   <u>Nori</u> - red algae; see brown algae.

C   <u>Nutmeg</u> - see mace/nutmeg.

X   <u>Nutrasweet</u> - 11; see aspartame.

C   <u>Nutrient additives</u> - nutrients added to mostly refined and processed foods giving a false sense of nutritional value and can lead to nutritional imbalances; chemicals used in preparing nutrients added are not listed on the label.

C A   <u>Oat gum</u> - 7, 46, 51; may cause gastrointestinal distress.

C   <u>Oil of caraway</u> - 9; see d-carvone.

C   <u>Oil of cloves</u> - 27; may cause gastrointestinal irritation in lab animals.

C   <u>Oil of Mace</u> - see mace/nutmeg.

C   <u>Oil of Nutmeg</u> - see mace/nutmeg.

* C   <u>Oil of rue</u> - 27; may cause photosensitivity; not adequately studied for carcinogenic effects.

X   <u>Olean</u> - see olestra.

* C   <u>Oleic acid</u> - 5, 12, 24; skin irritant, low oral

toxicity.

X   <u>Olestra</u> - 21; causes gastrointestinal irritation, reduces carotenoids and fat soluble vitamins in the body.

* S   <u>Oligofructose</u> – dietary fiber; prebiotic; health promoting benefits for the intestinal tract; largte amounts may cause flatulence or gastrointestinal distress.

* S   <u>Ox bile extract</u>

* C A   <u>Oxystearin</u> - 17; may be soy based; may have caused tumors in lab animals.

C A   <u>PABA</u> - see para aminobenzoic acid.

C   <u>Palm kernel oil</u> - see coconut oil.

S   <u>Pantothenic acid</u> - vitamin B5; see nutrient additives.

* C A   <u>Papain</u> - 15, 35; avoid if have ulcers; inhibits digestion if taken raw and in large doses.

* C   <u>Paprika, paprika oleoresin</u> - 38; may be harmful in large amounts.

C A   <u>Para aminobenzoic acid</u> - may cause light sensitivity, rash, swelling when applied to skin in sensitive individuals.

C A   <u>Parabens</u> - 6, 40; avoid if aspirin sensitive; not adequately tested.

C A   <u>Partially hydrogenated vegetable oil</u> - see hydrogenated vegetable oil.

C   <u>Pea protein</u> – contains high levels of glutamic acid; see free glutamates.

* S A   <u>Peanut oil</u> – cold pressed peanut oil may contain traces of peanut protein and is unsafe for those with peanut allergies; highly refined peanut oil does not contain traces of peanut protein and is safe for those with peanut allergies, however, highly refined oils are not healthy oil choices; those with peanut allergies should choose cold pressed, non-peanut oils.

C   <u>Pear oil</u> - see amyl acetate.

* C   <u>Pectins</u> - 19, 46, 51; commercially prepared pectins may be prepared with ammonia; may contain free glutamates; may cause flatulence, bloating; see MSG.

C   <u>PEG</u> – see polyethylene glycol.

* S   <u>Peptones</u> - 46.

C   <u>PGPR</u> – see polyglycerol polyricinoleic acid.

C   <u>Phenylalanine</u> – avoid if phenylketonuric; component of aspartame; listing this on the label may be a way of hiding aspartame; see aspartame.

X   <u>Phenylmethyl cyclosiloxane</u> - 4; have caused liver, kidney, reproductive damage in lab animals.

X   <u>Phenylpropanolamine</u> – causes headaches, increased blood pressure, strokes and death; women 18-49 at risk of hemorrhagic stroke.

C   <u>Phosphates</u> - 1, 19, 44, 50; can inhibit mineral absorption; excess consumption can cause kidney damage, osteoporosis.

* C <u>Phosphoric acid</u> - 1, 44; see phosphates.

S <u>Phylloquinone</u> - vitamin K1; see nutrient additives.

S <u>Phytonadione</u> - vitamin K1; see nutrient additives.

* C <u>Piperonal</u> - 9; chemical used to kill lice.

C <u>Plant sterol esters</u> – infants, children, pregnant and lactating women should avoid; those using cholesterol medication should seek advice from their doctor before using; not studied for effects of long-term usage.

C A <u>Polydextrose</u> - 11; may be corn based; may cause gastrointestinal distress; laxative effect.

C <u>Polyethylene glycol</u> – skin and eye irritant; slightly toxic when ingested; potential mutagen; may be contaminated with carcinogen 1,4-dioxane; can break down into formaldehyde.

C <u>Polyglycerol polyricinoleic acid</u> – 19; fatty acid ester of castor oil used mostly in chocolate; inadequate data on safety available.

C A <u>Polyoxyethylene-40-monostearate</u> - 5, 19; not adequately tested.

C A <u>Polyoxyethylene stearate</u> - 50; may cause gastrointestinal upset, skin rashes, kidney problems; chemically modified mono- & diglycerides.

C A   <u>Polysorbate 60</u> – 19; may be contaminated with a carcinogen.

C A   <u>Polysorbate 80</u> – see polysorbate 60.

C A   <u>Polysorbates</u> - 5, 19; sorbitol and corn, peanuts or soy based; possible contamination with a carcinogen.

X A   <u>Ponceau 4R</u> – coal tar dye; carcinogen.

C   <u>Potassium acetate</u> - may cause kidney problems.

* C1   <u>Potassium acid tartrate</u> - see cream of tartar.

* C1   <u>Potassium alginate</u> - 46, 51; avoid if pregnant, kidney or heart problems.

* C A   <u>Potassium benzoate</u> - may cause skin rashes, gastrointestinal upset; avoid if kidney, liver, heart problems.

* C1   <u>Potassium bicarbonate</u> - 33; see nutrient additives; avoid if kidney or heart problems.

X A   <u>Potassium bisulfite</u> - 6; see sodium bisulfite.

X   <u>Potassium bromate</u> - 34; can cause nervous system, kidney disorders, gastrointestinal upset; causes cancer in animals; banned worldwide except Japan and the U.S.

* C1   <u>Potassium carbonate</u> - 2; see nutrient additives; skin irritant; avoid if kidney or heart problems.

C A   <u>Potassium caseinate</u> - 50; avoid if kidney or heart problems; see caseinates.

* C   <u>Potassium chloride</u> - 43; see nutrient additives; can cause nausea, gastrointestinal irritation; caution if kidney, liver or heart problems.

* C A	<u>Potassium citrate</u> - 1, 7, 14, 44; see nutrient additives; may cause mouth ulcers; avoid if kidney or heart problems.
C1A	<u>Potassium fumarate</u> - 1; may be corn based; avoid if kidney or heart problems.
* C1A	<u>Potassium gluconate</u> - 14, 23, 26, 44; see nutrient additives; may be corn based; avoid if kidney or heart problems.
* C A	<u>Potassium glutamate</u> - 26; see MSG.
* S	<u>Potassium glycerophosphate</u> - see nutrient additives.
* C	<u>Potassium hydroxide</u> - may cause mouth ulcers, gastrointestinal upset.
* C1	<u>Potassium iodate</u> - 4, 18; caution if kidney, heart or thyroid problems.
* C1	<u>Potassium iodide</u> - see potassium iodate.
* S A	<u>Potassium lactate</u> - 27; see lactic acid.
X A	<u>Potassium metabisulfite</u> - 6; see sodium bisulfite.
X	<u>Potassium nitrate</u> - 6, 16; see nitrates.
X	<u>Potassium nitrite</u> - 6, 16; see nitrites.
* C	<u>Potassium phosphate</u> - 52; avoid if kidney, heart problems; see phosphates.
C	<u>Potassium polyphosphate</u> - may cause gastrointestinal upset; avoid if kidney or heart problems.
X A	<u>Potassium prosulfite</u> - see sodium bisulfite.
* C1	<u>Potassium sorbate</u> - 6, 40; avoid if kidney or heart problems; see sorbic acid.

* C   <u>Potassium sulfate</u> - may cause mouth ulcers, burning sensation in mouth.

  X A   <u>Potassium sulfite</u> - 3, 7, 40; see sodium bisulfite.

  X   <u>PPA</u> – see phenylpropanolamine.

  X A   <u>Processed free glutamic acid</u> – glutamic acid that has been manufactured and contains both d-glutamic and l-glutamic acid. L-glutamic acid, as found in protein and the human body, is bound to other amino acids in long chains and causes no adverse reactions. D-glutamic acid occurs as a result of the manufacturing process. It is a neurotoxin and causes brain lesions and neuroendocrine disorders in lab animals. In humans, it causes a great many symptoms, including skin rashes, tachycardia, migraine headaches, depression, and seizures. See MSG, free glutamates.

* C   <u>Propane</u> - 41; may be narcotic in high doses.

* C A   <u>Propionic acid</u> - 6; may trigger behavior changes.

* X A   <u>Propyl gallate</u> - 7; associated with kidney, liver problems, gastrointestinal irritation; suspected carcinogen; not adequately tested.

* X A   <u>Propylene glycol</u> - 24, 32, 50; "antifreeze;" skin and eye irritant, has caused nervous system and kidney damage in animals; ingestion can cause blindness, kidney failure, convulsions and death.

* X A   <u>Propylene glycol alginate</u> - 5, 46, 51; avoid if pregnant; see propylene glycol.

* X   <u>Propylene glycol monostearate</u> - 18, 19; may be corn, peanut, soy based; combined with hydrogenated vegetable oil.

* C A   <u>Propylparaben</u> - 6, 40; see parabens.

* S   <u>Pyridoxine hydrochloride</u> - vitamin B6; see nutrient additives.

   C   <u>Pyrophosphate</u> – 27; skin and mucous membrane irritant; has caused death in lab animals at low doses.

* S   <u>Quicklime</u> - 1, 18, 52; calcium oxide.

   X A   <u>Quinine</u> - 27; may impair hearing, cause birth defects; very poorly tested.

   C A   <u>Quorn</u> – see mycoprotein.

* X   <u>Rapeseed oil</u> – 19, 46; toxic; shown to cause lung cancer; may cause loss of vision, central nervous system disturbances, anemia, constipation, heart disease, low-birth-weight infants, irritability, respiratory problems or cancer.

* C   <u>Red algae</u> - see brown algae.

   X A   <u>Red No. 3</u> - 10; see FD&C Red No. 3.

   C A   <u>Red No. 40</u> - 10; see FD&C Red No. 40.

* C1A   <u>Reduced lactose whey</u> - avoid if milk allergies.

* C1A   <u>Reduced minerals whey</u> - avoid if milk allergies.

* S   <u>Rennet</u> - 20.

* S   <u>Riboflavin</u> - vitamin B2; see nutrient additives.

* S   <u>Riboflavin-5-phosphate</u> - vitamin B2; see nutrient additives.

   S   <u>Rice amasake</u> - 49; 1 Tbsp. contains 2 grams of sugars.

S   <u>Rice syrup</u> - 49; see barley malt.

S   <u>Rice syrup powder</u> - 49; 1 Tbsp. contains 4 grams of sugars; has some minerals and complex carbohydrates; all sweeteners are best avoided; see sucrose.

* C   <u>Rue</u> - see oil of rue.

X   <u>Saccharin</u> - 11; delisted as a carcinogen in 1997, however, studies still show that saccharin causes cancer.

* C   <u>Saffron</u> - 38; may be harmful in large amounts; not adequately tested.

C1   <u>Sage</u> – avoid if pregnant, epileptic or high blood pressure.

* C A   <u>St. John's bread gum</u> - locust bean gum.

C   <u>Salatrim</u> - 21; may cause nausea and stomach cramps; not adequately tested; not FDA approved.

C A   <u>Salicylates</u> - avoid if aspirin sensitive.

* C   <u>Salt</u> - see sodium chloride.

* C   <u>SAPP</u> - see sodium acid pyrophosphate.

C   <u>Selenium</u> – trace mineral essential for health; toxic if taken in excess.

C   <u>Silica</u> - 4; may be associated with kidney problems.

* C   <u>Silica aerogel</u> - 4; see silica.

C   <u>Silicates</u> - 4; see silica.

* C   <u>Silicon dioxide</u> - 4; see silica.

C   <u>Silicones</u> - 5; may be associated with kidney problems.

C   <u>Simplesse</u> - 21; not adequately tested.

C   <u>Smoked flavoring</u> - not adequately tested; may be carcinogenic.

C   <u>Smoked yeast</u> - not adequately tested; questionable safety.

* C   <u>Sodium acetate</u> - 14, 40; may cause blood pressure, kidney disturbances, water retention.

* C   <u>Sodium acid phosphate</u> - 44; see sodium acid pyrophosphate.

* C   <u>Sodium acid pyrophosphate</u> - 14, 33; skin, eye and respiratory irritant; can inhibit mineral absorption; may cause blood pressure, kidney disturbances, water retention; not adequately tested.

* C   <u>Sodium alginate</u> - 17, 46, 51; may cause blood pressure, kidney disturbances, pregnancy complications.

* C   <u>Sodium aluminum phosphate</u> - see aluminum, sodium acid pyrophosphate.

C   <u>Sodium aluminum sulfate</u> - 13, 34; causes kidney failure in lab animals; see aluminum, sodium acetate.

* C   <u>Sodium aluminosilicate</u> - 4; may be associated with kidney problems, mineral malabsorption.

* C A   <u>Sodium ascorbate</u> - 7; see nutrient additives; synthetic vitamin C; may be corn based; may

contribute to blood pressure, kidney
disturbances, water retention.

* C A   <u>Sodium benzoate</u> - 6, 40; see benzoate of soda.
* C   <u>Sodium bicarbonate</u> - 14, 33; baking soda; see
sodium acetate.
  X A   <u>Sodium bisulfite</u> - 3, 6, 7; destroys vitamin B1;
small amounts may cause asthma, anaphylactic
shock; dangerous for asthma, allergy sufferers;
has caused deaths; banned on fresh fruits and
vegetables, except potatoes.
* C   <u>Sodium calcium aluminosilicate</u> - 4; may be
associated with kidney problems, mineral
malabsorption.
* C   <u>Sodium carboxymethylcellulose</u> - 4, 17, 51;
causes cancer in animals; may contribute to
blood pressure, kidney and digestive
disturbances, water retention; not adequately
tested.
* C   <u>Sodium carbonate</u> - 39; may cause heart
problems, gastrointestinal distress; see sodium
acetate.
* C A   <u>Sodium caseinate</u> - 50; avoid if milk allergy or
MSG sensitive; may contain free glutamates; see
sodium ascorbate, MSG, casein.
* C   <u>Sodium chloride</u> - 26, 40; may cause blood
pressure, kidney disturbances, water retention.
* C   <u>Sodium citrate</u> - 1, 7, 14, 19, 27, 44; see sodium
acetate, citric acid.

X A   Sodium cocoyl glutamate – see glutamates.

* C   Sodium diacetate - 6; see sodium acetate.

* C A   Sodium erythorbate - 7; may be corn based; see sodium ascorbate.

   C   Sodium ferrocyanide - 4; see sodium acetate.

   C   Sodium formate - may cause urinary tract problems.

   C A   Sodium fumarate - 1; may be corn based; see sodium ascorbate.

* C A   Sodium gluconate - 44; see sodium ascorbate.

* C   Sodium hexametaphosphate - 19, 44, 46, 51; see sodium acid pyrophosphate.

   X A   Sodium hydrosulfite - see sodium bisulfite.

* C   Sodium hydroxide - 2, 39; caustic soda, lye; alters protein content of food; see sodium acetate.

* C A   Sodium isoascorbate - see sodium ascorbate.

* C   Sodium lactate - 7, 23, 32; see sodium acetate.

   C A   Sodium lauryl sulfate - skin, eye, mucous membrane irritant; skin contact may cause allergic reactions; moderately toxic if ingested; may cause mutagenic effects.

   X A   Sodium metabisulfite - see sodium bisulfite.

* C   Sodium metaphosphate - 18, 44; see sodium acid pyrophosphate.

* C   Sodium metasilicate - see silica, sodium acid pyrophosphate.

   X   Sodium nitrate - see nitrates.

X   <u>Sodium nitrite</u> - see nitrites.

* C   <u>Sodium pantothenate</u> - see nutrient additives, sodium acetate.

* C   <u>Sodium pectinate</u> - 46, 51; see sodium acetate.

* C   <u>Sodium phosphate</u> - 44; see sodium acid pyrophosphate.

C   <u>Sodium polyphosphate</u> - may cause gastrointestinal upset; see sodium acid pyrophosphate.

* C   <u>Sodium potassium tartrate</u> - 1, 19; may cause blood pressure, kidney disturbances; avoid if heart problems.

* C A   <u>Sodium propionate</u> – 6, 40; may trigger headaches, behavioral changes, blood pressure, kidney disturbances, water retention.

* C   <u>Sodium pyrophosphate</u> - 44; see sodium acid pyrophosphate.

S   <u>Sodium riboflavin phosphate</u> - vitamin B2; see nutrient additives.

C   <u>Sodium selenite</u> – form of selenium often found in nutritional supplements; safe at less than 600 mcg/day for adults, individual needs vary, see your healthcare provider to determine your individual needs; toxic if taken in excess; see selenium.

* C   <u>Sodium sesquicarbonate</u> - 39; see sodium acetate.

* C   <u>Sodium silicate</u> - 4; see sodium acetate.

C	<u>Sodium silicoaluminate</u> - 4; see sodium calcium aluminosilicate.
* C	<u>Sodium sorbate</u> - 3, 6; may cause blood pressure, kidney, liver disturbances, water retention.
C A	<u>Sodium stearoyl fumarate</u> - 18, 19; may be corn, milk, peanut, soy based; see sodium acetate, stearic acid.
C A	<u>Sodium stearoyl lactylate</u> - 18, 19, 46; see sodium stearoyl fumarate.
C	<u>Sodium sulfate</u> - 14; may cause heart, kidney problems; see sodium acetate.
* X A	<u>Sodium sulfite</u> - 3, 6, 40; see sodium bisulfite.
C A	<u>Sodium sulfoacetate mono- & diglycerides</u> - 19; not adequately tested.
* C	<u>Sodium tartrate</u> - 1, 19; see sodium acetate.
* C	<u>Sodium thiosulfate</u> - 7; see sodium acetate.
* C	<u>Sodium tripolyphosphate</u> – 40, 44, 46, 50, 51; can cause calcium depletion; skin and mucous membrane irritant; may cause violent vomiting or diarrhea if ingested; GRAS for packaging.
C	<u>Softeners</u> - see ester gum.
* C	<u>Sorbic acid</u> - 3,6, 40; may cause skin rashes; interferes with enzyme functions in the body; has caused cancer in lab animals; mildly toxic when ingested; mutagen.
C A	<u>Sorbitan monopalmitate</u> - 19; see polysorbates.
C A	<u>Sorbitan monostearate</u> - 5, 19, 46; see polysorbates, stearic acid.

C A   <u>Sorbitan tristearate</u> - 19; see polysorbates, stearic acid.

* C A   <u>Sorbitol</u> - 11; may cause extreme gastrointestinal distress, bloating, diarrhea, abdominal pain, especially in infants and children; DO NOT give to infants and children; may be corn based.

C   <u>Sorghum molasses</u> - 49; see sucrose.

S   <u>Sorghum syrup</u> - 49; see barley malt.

C   <u>Soy</u> – contains toxins that cannot be completely removed with processing, enzyme inhibitors that block enzymes needed for digestion, phytates that inhibit mineral absorption; promotes clumping of red blood cells, kidney stones; depresses thyroid function; weakens immune system; fermented soy products have less toxins.

C A   <u>Soy concentrates</u> - 22; see soy isolates, free glutamates, MSG.

* C A   <u>Soy isolates</u> - 22; may inhibit nutrient absorption; may be contaminated with nitrites; see free glutamates, MSG.

C A   <u>Soy oil</u> – contaminated with hexane from chemical extraction at high temperatures; may be genetically modified.

C A   <u>Spice</u> - generic term to protect trade secrets; may be a combination of many different spices; may be fumigated or irradiated.

C   <u>Splenda</u> – see sucralose.

* C   <u>Stannous chloride</u> - 7; skin and mucous

membrane irritant; not adequately tested.

* C A   <u>Starch</u> - 51; may be corn, wheat based; see modified food starch.

* C   <u>Starter distillate</u> - 9; see diacetyl.

* C   <u>Stearic acid</u> - 5, 12; may be derived from hydrogenated oils.

C A   <u>Stearoyl lactylate</u> – 18, 19; see calcium stearoyl lactylate, sodium stearoyl lactylate.

C A   <u>Stearoyl propylene glycol hydrogen succinate</u> - 19; see propylene glycol, stearic acid.

C A   <u>Stearoyls</u> - 18, 19; may be corn, milk, peanut, soy based; see stearic acid.

* C A   <u>Stearyl citrate</u> - 7, 44; may be corn based; see stearic acid, calcium citrate.

C   <u>Stellar</u> - 21; not adequately tested.

* C   <u>Sterculia gum</u> - see vegetable gum.

S   <u>Stevia</u> - 49; can be used by those with candida, diabetes, hypoglycemia.

* C   <u>STPP</u> – see sodium tripolyphosphate.

S A   <u>Sucanat</u> - 49; 1 Tbsp. contains 3 grams of sugars; all sweeteners are best avoided; see sucrose.

* C   <u>Succinic acid</u> - 14, 27, 39; laxative effect.

C A   <u>Succistearin</u> - 19; see stearoyl propylene glycol hydrogen succinate.

C   <u>Sucralite</u> – see sucralose

C   <u>Sucralose</u> - 11; chlorinated sugar; contrary to manufacturer's claims, sucralose is partially absorbed and metabolized by the body, 11-27%

according to the FDA and 40% according to the Japanese Food Sanitation Council; has caused shrunken thymus gland, enlarged liver and kidneys; miscarriage, diarrhea in animal studies; contains small amounts of dangerous contaminants, such as heavy metals, methanol, arsenic, triphenilphosphine oxide, chlorinated disaccharides, chlorinated monosaccharides; no independient studies on effects on humans or studies for long-term effects in humans; no monitoring of adverse health effects; those with chlorine allergies may suffer severe reactions.

* C   Sucrose - 49; associated with blood sugar problems, depression, fatigue, B-vitamin deficiency, hyperactivity, tooth decay, periodontal disease, indigestion.

C   Sucrose polyester - 21; not adequately tested.

C   Sugar - see sucrose.

C   Sugar alcohols - mannitol, sorbitol, xylitol, lactitol, isomalt, maltitol, erythritol and hydrogenated starch hydrolysates; may cause laxative effect, bloating, diarrhea; may cause carbohydrate cravings

X   Sulfites - see sodium bisulfite.

* X   Sulfur dioxide - 3, 7, 40; see sodium bisulfite.

X   Sweet 'n Low - 11; contains saccharin.

* C   Talc - may contain asbestos contamination.

* C   Tagatose – 11; may cause nausea, flatulence, diarrhea.
* C   Tallow - may contribute to heart disease.
* C   Tannic acid - 15, 27; may be carcinogenic.
* C   Tannin - see tannic acid.
* S   Tartaric acid - 1; may cause gastrointestinal distress.
  C A   Tartrazine - 10; FD&C Yellow No. 5; may cause breathing difficulty, hay fever, skin rashes, blurred vision; avoid if aspirin sensitive.
  S   Taurine - amino acid; see nutrient additives.
  C   TBHQ - 7; questionable safety; not adequately tested.
  C   Tertiary butylhydroquinone - see TBHQ.
* X   Tetrasodium pyrophosphate – 19, 44; poison if ingested; can cause nausea, vomiting, diarrhea; GRAS for packaging.
  C A   Textured vegetable protein (TVP) - 22; chemically processed; may contain free glutamates; see MSG.
  C   THBP - 7; questionable safety; not adequately tested.
* S   Thiamine hydrochloride - synthetic vitamin B1; see nutrient additives.
* S   Thiamine mononitrate - synthetic vitamin B1; see nutrient additives.
* S   Thiodipropionic acid - 7, 40.
* S A   Thyme oil - 27.

φ C   Titanium dioxide – 38; may irritate skin; inhalation of large amounts of titanium dioxide dust may cause lung damage; use limited to 1% by weight; inadequate information available to determine if carcinogenic to humans.

* S A   Tocopherol - 7; vitamin E; see nutrient additives; may be corn, peanut, soy based.

* C A   Tragacanth - 46, 51; can cause gastrointestinal distress; not adequately tested.

* C   Trehalose – 46, 49; may cause gastrointestinal distress when consumed in large amounts.

* C   Triacetin - see glyceryl triacetate.

* C   Tribasic calcium phosphate - see calcium phosphate.

* C   Tribasic potassium phosphate - see potassium phosphate.

* C   Tricalcium phosphate - see calcium phosphate.

* C   Tricalcium silicate - 4; see silicates.

* S A   Triethyl citrate - 44; may interfere with medical lab test results.

C   2-4-5 Trihydroxybutrophenone - see THBP.

* C A   Tripotassium citrate - see potassium citrate.

* C   Trisodium phosphate - 44, 50; see sodium acid pyrophosphate.

* X   TSPP – see tetrasodium pyrophosphate.

* C   Tumeric - 38; may be extracted with harmful solvents.

* C   Turmeric - same as tumeric.

S	<u>Urea</u>
* C	<u>Vanillin</u> - 9; see ethyl vanillin.
C	<u>Vegetable broth</u> - 27; may contain additives not listed on the label.
C A	<u>Vegetable gum</u> - 19, 46, 51; not adequately tested.
C	<u>Vegetable oil sterols</u> – see plant sterol esters.
C	<u>Vegetable shortening</u> - generally is saturated fat or hydrogenated oil; associated with cardiovascular disease.
C	<u>Veratraldehyde</u> - 26; see ethyl vanillin.
* S	<u>Vitamin A</u> - dietary supplement; may be toxic in very large doses; see nutrient additives.
* S	<u>Vitamin A acetate</u> - synthetic vitamin A; may be toxic in very large doses; see nutrient additives.
* S	<u>Vitamin A palmitate</u> - synthetic vitamin A; may be toxic in very large doses; see nutrient additives.
* S	<u>Vitamin B1</u> - dietary supplement; see nutrient additives.
* S	<u>Vitamin B2</u> - dietary supplement; see nutrient additives.
* S	<u>Vitamin B3</u> - dietary supplement; see nutrient additives.
* S	<u>Vitamin B6</u> - dietary supplement; see nutrient additives.
* S	<u>Vitamin B12</u> - dietary supplement; see nutrient additives.

* S   <u>Vitamin C</u> - dietary supplement; see nutrient additives.
* S   <u>Vitamin D2</u> - synthetic vitamin D; may be toxic in very large doses; see nutrient additives.
* S   <u>Vitamin D3</u> - natural vitamin D; may be toxic in very large doses; see nutrient additives.
  S   <u>Vitamin G</u> - vitamin B2; see nutrient additives.
  S A   <u>Wheat bran</u>
  S A   <u>Wheat germ</u>
* C1A   <u>Wheat gluten</u> - 18; avoid if gluten sensitive or malabsorption syndrome.
* C1A   <u>Whey</u> - 12; avoid if lactose intolerance or milk allergies.
  C A   <u>Whey protein</u> – see free glutamates.
* C A   <u>Whey protein concentrate</u> - may contain free glutamates see soy isolates, MSG, whey.
* C A   <u>White thyme oil</u> - 27; may cause gastrointestinal upset, dizziness, cardiac depression.
  X   <u>Wormwood</u> - 27; see artemisia.
  C A   <u>Xanthan gum</u> - 48, 51; may cause gastrointestinal distress; extracted from Xanthomonas campestris by solvent extraction which may leave a toxic residue; may contain allowable amounts of lead, arsenic and heavy metals.
  C   <u>Xylitol</u> - 11; 20-28 grams per day can be safely used for those weighing more than 100 lbs.; limit children to 1-2 grams/10 pounds of body weight/day; high doses may cause

gastrointestinal distress; has caused cancer in lab animals at high doses.

C A   <u>Yeast autolyzates</u> - may contain free glutamates; not adequately tested; see MSG.

C A   <u>Yeast-malt sprout extract</u> - 26; may contain free glutamates; see MSG.

C A   <u>Yellow No. 5</u> - 10; see FD&C Yellow No. 5.

X A   <u>Yellow No. 6</u> - 10; see FD&C Yellow No. 6.

C   <u>Yellow prussiate of soda</u> - 4; see sodium ferrocyanide.

* S A   <u>Zein</u> - corn protein.

* S   <u>Zinc chloride</u> - see nutrient additives; excess can cause anemia, gastrointestinal distress, mild skin irritation.

* S   <u>Zinc gluconate</u> - see nutrient additives, zinc chloride.

S   <u>Zinc methionine sulfate</u> - see nutrient additives, zinc chloride.

* S   <u>Zinc oxide</u> - see nutrient additives, zinc chloride.

* C   <u>Zinc stearate</u> - see nutrient additives, zinc chloride, stearic acid.

* C   <u>Zinc sulfate</u> - see nutrient additives; excess can cause anemia, gastrointestinal distress, mild skin irritation; has caused tumors in lab animals.

REFERENCES

A. Branen, P. Davidson, S. Salminen, FOOD ADDITIVES. New York: Marcel Dekker, Inc., 1990.

Center for Science in the Public Interest, http://www.cspinet.org/reports/chemcuisine.htm.

Nicholas Freydberg, Ph.D. and Willis A. Gortner, Ph.D., THE FOOD ADDITIVES BOOK. New York: Bantam Books, 1982.

Ann Louise Gittleman, GET THE SUGAR OUT: 501 Simple Ways To Cut The Sugar Out Of Any Diet. New York: Crown Trade Paperbacks, 1996.

Mark Gold, Aspartame/NutraSweet Toxicity Info Center http://www.holisticmed.com/aspartame/

Nikki & David Goldbeck, THE GOLDBECK'S GUIDE TO GOOD FOOD. New York: New American Library, 1987.

Robert Goodman, A QUICK GUIDE TO FOOD SAFETY. San Diego: Silvercat Publications, 1992.

HEALTH ALERT Newsletter.

Grace Ross Lewis, 1001 CHEMICALS IN EVERYDAY PRODUCTS. John Wiley & Sons, 1999.

Dr. Joseph Mercola http://www.mercola.com/2000/dec/3/sucralose_dangers.htm

Earl Mindell, UNSAFE AT ANY MEAL. New York: Warner Books, 1987.

Bill Misner, Ph.D., Xylitol research, Director of Research & Product Development E-CAPS INC. & HAMMER NUTRITION LIMITED

Jack L. Samuels, Truth in Labeling Campaign, http://www.truthinlabeling.org

Doris Sarjeant & Karen Evans, HARD TO SWALLOW: The Truth About Food Additives. Canada: Alive Books, 1999.

David Steinman & Samuel S. Epstein, M.D., THE SAFE SHOPPER'S BIBLE. New York: MacMillan, 1995.

Ruth Winter, A CONSUMER'S DICTIONARY OF FOOD ADDITIVES. New York: Crown Publishers, 1999.

Ruth Winter, POISONS IN YOUR FOOD. New York: Crown Publishers, 1991.

At KISS For Health, our mission is to provide the highest quality and safest health and nutrition products and information available. We search the marketplace to find products that meet up to our "highest quality" standards.

Information on KISS For Health books can be found on the web at:

http://www.kiss4healthpublishing.com
http://www.healthyeatingadvisor.com/foodadditives.html
http://www.healthyeatingadvisor.com/healthyeating.html

The Healthy Eating Advisor has an abundance of healthy eating information and links to healthy products and other healthy websites.

http://www.healthyeatingadvisor.com

These websites offer healthy products at wholesale prices:

http://www.nomorecandida.com
http://www.globalhealthtrax.org/drfarlow
http://healthy4life.themastersmiracle.com
(You can order wholesale or retail here.)

Books By This Author

DYING TO LOOK GOOD: The Disturbing Truth About What's Really in Your Cosmetics, Toiletries and Personal Care Products
$10.95 + $3.00 S&H + 7.75% tax (CA residents)

FOOD ADDITIVES: A Shopper's Guide To What's Safe & What's Not
$4.95 + $1.50 S&H + 7.75% tax (CA residents)

HEALTHY EATING: For Extremely Busy People Who Don't Have Time For It.
$7.95 + $3.00 S&H + 7.75% tax (CA residents)

Books by this author may be ordered from KISS For Health Publishing. Payment accepted by check, money order, phone check or fax check (U.S. funds only):

KISS For Health Publishing
PO Box 462335-C
Escondido, CA 92046-2335
Tel. (760) 735-8101 • Fax (760) 746-8937
e-mail: kiss4health@lycos.com

Excerpts, information on the contents of these books and reviews may be found on Amazon.com,
http://www.kiss4healthpublishing.com
http://www.healthyeatingadvisor.com/foodadditives.html
http://www.healthyeatingadvisor.com/healthyeating.html

Order Form

Qty	Title	Price
	DYING TO LOOK GOOD ($10.95 ea)	
	FOOD ADDITIVES ($4.95 ea)	
	HEALTHY EATING ($7.95 ea)	
S&H **(U.S.)**	DYING TO LOOK GOOD $3.00 FOOD ADDITIVES $1.50 HEALTHY EATING $3.00 Multiple copies - $3.00 for 1st book, $1.00 for each additional book	
Subtotal		
Tax (CA residents 7.75%)		
Total		

Send check or money order (U.S. funds only) to:

KISS For Health Publishing • PO Box 462335-C
Escondido, CA 92046-2335

To pay by phone or fax check, or for contact
information for non U.S. shipping rates, see page 79.